DIY Aromatherapy: The Best Beginner's Step-By-Step Guide to Essential Oils and Aromatherapy Secrets – Recipes Included

DISCLAIMER:

This book has been written for the benefit of the readers who are interested in the healing power of Aromatherapy. Anyone who is interested in using this form of treatment is encouraged to read this book to learn more about aromatherapy.

The guide gives a detailed overview about this alternative medicine as well as a brief history about how this form of treatment has come about. This has gone through thorough research and has passed the standards needed. We also keep updated information about the topic that is discussed on this guide.

However, we do not claim that the things that are written here are 100% effective and it is still important to seek medical advice before trying aromatherapy. This is to ensure that you will really benefit to the programs under this.

We also do not promote the use of any products that are used to day for aromatherapy. This is the reason why you should act with discernment and choose the best product that suits you.

No part of this guide should be reproduced without permission from the owners of the book.

Table of Contents

SUMMARY:

This is a detailed guide on everything you need to know about aromatherapy and the products that are available in the market. We have all the things you'll need to know about aromatherapy as well as the various essential and carrier oils.

Most of the contents of this guide will teach you how to use these essential oils for therapy. This includes important facts on how to apply this to your body as well as how these oils are extracted and mixed with carrier oil.

Aside from that, this guide will give you in-depth knowledge about everything there is when it comes to aromatherapy. Having this knowledge is very important because aromatherapy helps promote good health as well as benefit the body with the effects it has.

Aromatherapy has gained popularity over the years and has been proven to be an effective treatment to the body and soul. Check out the different oils in this guide to know more about the benefits of at this form of treatment.

The guide also speaks about other interesting things like the world of essential oils and the many benefits of these precious liquids to our body. There is also a page dedicated in discussing all about carrier oils as well as safety precautions when it comes to doing aromatherapy.

Introduction

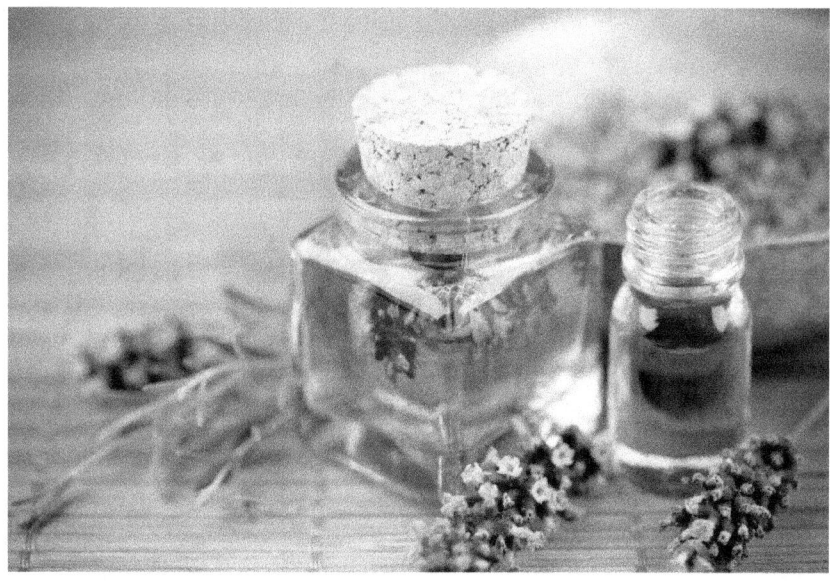

Have you ever tried to calm yourself with the use of some essential oils or scented candles purchased in the market? If yes, then you already tried aromatherapy which is a treatment used in taking care of some health problems that our body experience. This form of treatment uses essential oils from various plants to relieve a person from certain ailments.

This is another form of alternative medicine that uses oils derived from specific plants as well as other compounds that are considered as aroma therapeutic. These oils should have an altering effect on the mind, mood, physical or psychological well-being.

Aroma therapists are the ones who are responsible in making these essential oils. They have studied the different properties of these oils as well specialize in the use of these oils as treatment for certain ailments. They know how to use and apply this for the benefit of a person's health.

Most of the time, aromatherapy is used to relax both the mind and the body with the scents that are released and inhaled by our body. Its calming effect made it renowned around the world as a relaxant which helps a person to feel relieved after a long day's work.

However, aside from being a relaxant, there are other ailments that aromatherapy helps cure or at least correct. We would be discussing these benefits later on. We will first discuss the brief history of aromatherapy.

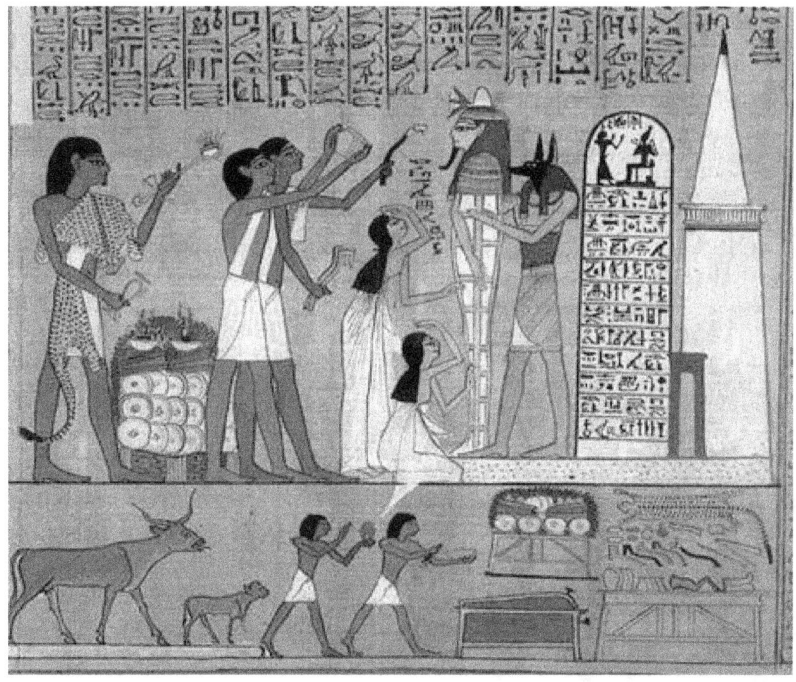

According to Anthropologists, the history of aromatherapy has already been used by ancient civilizations. The Egyptians are said to be the first civilization to use this method. Egyptian priests used to burn resins and gums for incense. They also burn bundles of aromatic plants and use this for the same purpose.

Take note, these priests also served as doctors during those times. They used the fragrant oils extracted from plants for both religious and magical ceremonies. They even use these extracts for embalming or some kind of offering to their deities.

Even the father of Modern Medicine, Hippocrates, recognizes the psychological and physical benefits of scented oils and ointments.

According to this pioneer, aromatic bath as well as scented massage is a key on having good health.

China and India also recognizes the use of aromatic oils during the time that Egypt is also using it. Ayurvedic medicine also promotes massage using aromatic oils. Roses during those times are deemed as effective antidepressants and were also believed to be effective in keeping the liver healthy. Studies today have proven that the essential oils that were promoted before are still effective to this day.

The Persians, however, are the ones that are given credited when we speak about distillation of these essential oils. There are other proofs though, that this process has been used long before this ancient civilization has started doing this during the 10th century.

From this information, we can now proceed to learn more about the process of obtaining essential oils which are used in aromatherapy. This involves the process mentioned above but it may also include other steps. Besides, there are other things to be considered to obtain this product and those who make this knows how delicate and complicated this process and can be.

What Are Essential Oils

Essential oils are products that are extracted from various plants and contain aroma compounds which benefit the body. Other terms used to call this product may be aetherolea, ethereal oils and volatile oils. We call these essential oils because they contain the "essence" of the plant to which they are extracted from.

The Process involved in obtaining essential oil requires distillation commonly with the use of steam. Other processes involve solvent extraction. There are several uses for essential oil which includes being an ingredient for several other products like perfumes, soaps, cosmetics, flavoring as well as household cleaning products. However, way before essential oils were used for these products, they've been used already for its medicinal properties and is noted for the way they treat several ailments.

You may be curious enough to wonder how essential oils are extracted from plants. Before discussing the direct processes that are involved in extracting this valuable liquid, we have provided an overview on how the whole process goes.

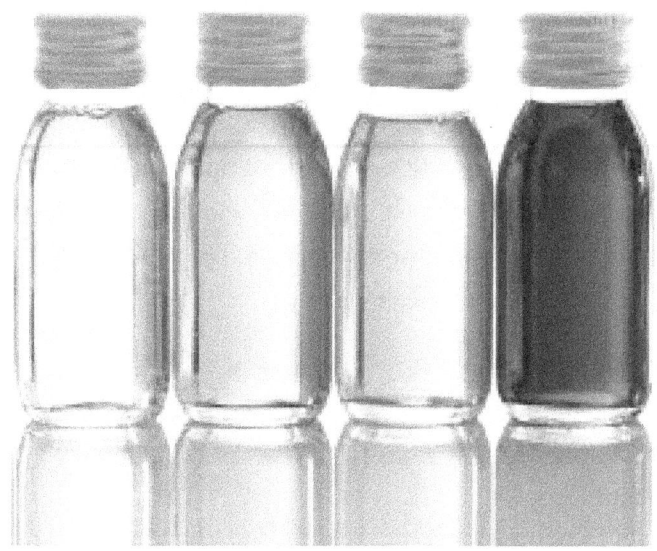

1. The first step involves extracting or harvesting the oil from the plant which will be used for the body. There are many plant materials that can be used for this purpose and we have included this in our guide.
2. In order for the extracted oil to work effectively and easily, this may be combined with carrier oil. It is important to use this kind of oil so it will remain intact and it also makes it easier to apply to your body.
3. There are other application methods that the oil can be added. One may choose to use this as a topical ointment or

use it or diffuse it in the air. Others massage this on the body to relieve ailments like backache.

4. After using these essential oils, you'll end up getting the many benefits of using this therapy. The aroma released from this oil is later gets into the body through inhaling it as well as penetrating to your pores.

PRODUCING ESSENTIAL OILS

This process may seem simple but extracting the oil itself is not that easy. As mentioned eariler, this product is extracted from plants and they don't come instantly like fruits or other products that are derived from plants.

Here are the things you need to know when it comes to obtaining these essential oils.

Distillation

Most essential oils are extracted with the use of distillation. As mentioned earlier, it may have begun years before it was recorded in Persia which means that extracting essential oils through this method started before the 10th century.

Deriving essential oils from plants like peppermint, lavender, eucalyptus involves distillation. These oils may come from the raw material from plants like leaves, flowers, bark, wood, seeds, roots, peel or their very seeds which are later put into a distillation apparatus called alembic with water already in it. The vapors go through a coil which will later condense and return to its liquid form. The liquid are collected on another vial.

Among all the essential oils that are made through this process, only ylang-ylang takes 22 hours to extract through fractional distillation since other oils require only a single process.

Solvent Extraction

Another process that is used in extracting essential oils is through solvent extraction. This requires adding a solvent to the raw plant material to extract these oils from air. Hexane is usually involved in this process to make it successful.

After this, a waxy material will be left behind after this is done. The term used for this material is concrete and is what will be used to obtain the oil. Ethyl alcohol will later be used to extract the oils from it.

Resins

There are some cases that resins are used in order to obtain the oil. This involvesmaterials that can be cooked or heated over herbal surface. The oils will later be obtained on the surface after the process is completed.

This is usually used to obtain oils that are difficult to extract. It may not be used on other herbs but only those that have been proven to be tough to obtain.

Carbon Dioxide

Another way of obtaining essential oils is by adding carbon dioxide which makes the process easier. The products produced using this gas are believed to be superior compared to the traditional means of extracting essential oils. It doesn't affect the quality of the oil.

The extraction process involves pumping pressurized carbon dioxide into a container with the raw plant material. Under these circumstances, Carbon dioxide now has liquid properties even if it still remains on its former state. The liquid serves as the solvent which pulls the oil and other materials into the plant matter.

THE DIFFERENT WAYS ON HOW TO BENEFIT FROM ESSENTIAL OILS

As part of aromatherapy, it is important to have knowledge on the different ways on how to use this product. This may involve different ways on how to use in order for your body to benefit from it. Here are the known ways on how to benefit from this product.

STEAM TREATMENT

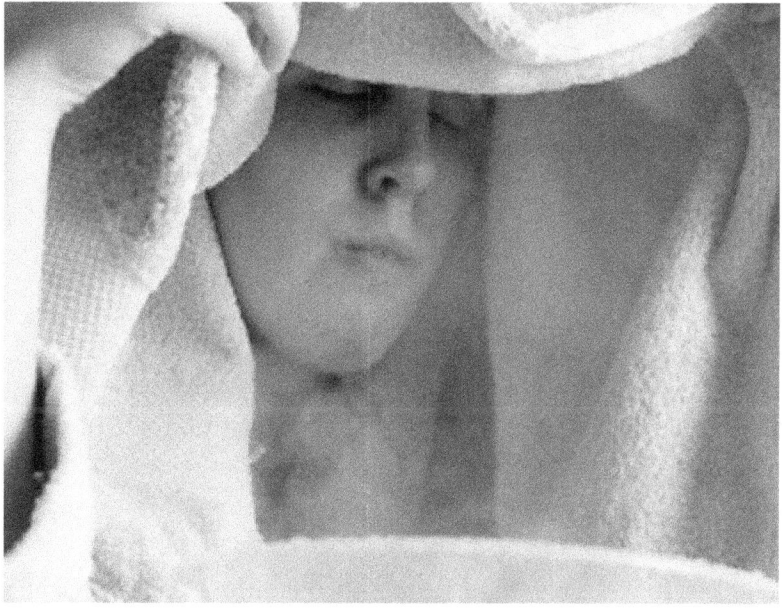

Using steam treatment is one of the most common ways of aromatherapy. If you choose to use this method, then you should have a diffuser. Steam is being used in the process in order to fill the place with aroma.

When doing this on a spa, it is recommended for the person to lie down in order to get the full benefits of this treatment.

Some of the benefits of steam therapy is as follows:

Weight loss

Detoxification

Relief for stress

Relief for allergies

Cellulite reduction

Effective relief for Joint pain

Relieves sore and tired muscles

Improves blood circulation

Reduces inflammation

Immunity booster

Interested in having your own steam therapy at home? Then here are the basic steps to follow. It's so easy that you'll find yourself relaxed in no time.

1. The first step is to add water into a diffuser or vaporizer which you add in your home. the design should allow you to relax your body.
2. Just add a few drops of the essential oil of your choice into a steam cleaner. All you need is just three to five drops of this oil.
3. When the water gets heated up, it will give off steam along with the oil that you have added.
4. Enjoy the relaxing scent of the oil while letting it pass through your airways.

This is so easy to use that you may even use a handheld vaporizer can be used. And if you will notice, all that is needed during a steam therapy is just a few drops of essential oils. Stronger amount of this can be dangerous. This product is dense that you don't need to overuse the product.

STEAM BATH

Others use essential oils on steam bath that there are individuals who have created their very own steam room inside their homes just for this purpose. A steam bath system allows those who want this to use these essential oils on steam showers.

There are several benefits of choosing steam bath and you might find this to be popular in Asian countries where it got its roots. The water doesn't need to be very hot but it should be warm enough to create steam.

You may wonder how to make your own steam bath and here are the few simple steps on how to make your own.

1. Combine between to five drops of essential oil to a few tablespoons of carrier oil. Add this mixture under tap in the tub. This is to spread the oil evenly throughout the place.
2. Make sure that the steam stays in the tub so it is advisable for you to close the area using either curtains or any other borders available.
3. Allow the steam to penetrate through the pores and take a deep breath every once in a while for you to take in the benefits into your body through your nostrils.
4. For best results, do this for ten to twenty minutes so that your body can benefit from the steam bath.

There are several benefits of having a steam bath which includes the following:

- Clears the mucus in your lungs
- Helps relieve respiratory infections
- Relieves asthma
- Helps cure bronchitis
- Clears the throat and avoids hoarseness
- It can also relieve allergies
- Reduces the symptoms of joint pain and arthritis
- Relieves muscle pain and muscle tension
- Helps overcome stress and anxiety
- Helps promote regular sleep
- Releases negative energies

According to studies, these essential oils are better than soap since it keeps the skin healthy. Sweating is said to be a good way to release all the toxins in the skin which results to having a healthier skin. Aside from that, it promotes better blood circulation on the blood vessels under the skin. It also opens up the pores and removes more dirt that is stuck inside. This is the reason why it is said that this can help cure or relieve the symptoms of the following skin diseases:

- Acne
- Eczema
- Chapped and dry skin

Aromatherapy massage

A good massage can bring a lot of benefits to your body. For one, you can immediately feel your tired muscles ease. However, if you add essential oils along with the massage, then you get more health benefits from the massage.

A few drops are all you'll need in order to benefit from these essential oils. Just add these drops on traditional massage oils and you are now ready to use it.

The process of using essential oil for aroma therapeutic massage involves only a few simple steps to follow. Read the ways on how to use essential oils for aroma therapeutic massage.

1. There will be a series of essential oils that will be used by massage therapist depending on your needs and where it will be applied. The oils are then mixed together on massage oil so it can be easily spread throughout the body.
2. First, the therapist will use gentle motions and strokes to massage the oil throughout the body. The oil will later be applied on the right area and later be stimulated through different strokes and movements that the massage therapist will use.

3. The massage therapist will then move his arms around the body for some time which depends on the part that should be treated.
4. The massage will last for as long as you need and depends on the condition of your body.

As good as it sounds; there are still necessary things to remember before deciding to go on an aroma therapeutic massage. Remember, the oil is applied directly on your skin and there are still several things to remember when it comes to applying this kind of liquid in the body.

1. Those who have open wounds are not allowed to have an aromatherapy massage since there is a high chance for infection.
2. Bruised spots (also known as closed wounds) should not receive massage as well.
3. Also, those who have had surgical procedures should not have a massage since it may stress the body since the body is not yet prepared for it.
4. Those cancer patients who just underwent radiation therapy or chemotherapy are not allowed to undergo aromatherapy unless the doctor allows this while the treatment is undergoing.
5. Since aromatherapy massage requires motions that may squeeze or press the skin, it is advisable for those who are prone to blood clots to avoid this as well.
6. It is also better to have a massage on empty stomach or just eating a few snacks before the treatment. This will help prevent the digestive tract from getting upset.

DIRECT CONTACT TO SKIN

The last method used in aromatherapy is applying the oil directly on the skin. Grab an essential oil that suits your preference.

1. The first step is to combine the essential oil of your choice with carrier oil. Dilute the essential oil so that the aroma won't be too strong for you.
2. Apply the mixed oil directly on the body on the spot that you want to cure.
3. Let the area dry off by itself after some time. It takes a little long for the oil to dry and penetrate into the skin. The aroma from the oil can also benefit you through inhaling it through your nasal passages. As soon as you do, you can feel more relaxed as you apply this on your body.

Just like massage, these essential oils are applied directly on skin so the reminder mentioned in the aromatherapy massage is also considered with this method. So before applying a mixture of essential oils and carrier oils on your skin, it is important to remember those things before applying it directly on skin.

If you are able to do this right, then you will surely benefit through this kind of alternative treatment. There are several advantages of aromatherapy and you may find a more comprehensive list of benefits aromatherapy for your body. You will be surprised that there are several things that you didn't know about this treatment and the next section of this guide will discuss the all the benefits aromatherapy has for your body and overall health.

HEALTH BENEFITS OF AROMATHERAPY FOR YOUR BODY

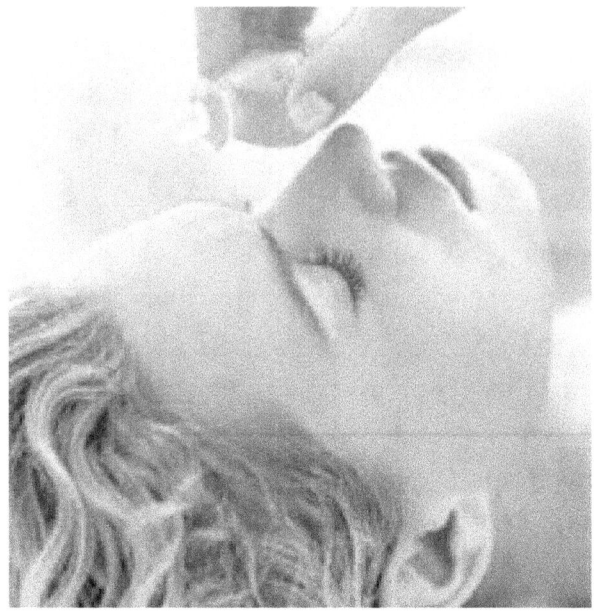

Aromatherapy has countless of benefits to your body and overall health. It affects almost all the systems of your body which is the reason why many individuals are now recognizing this kind of alternative treatment as the best way of relieving several ailments. Of course, medical opinion from medical practitioners and family doctors is still important before indulging in this relaxing treatment.

Health Benefits for the Muscular system

The first thing that will come to mind when we think about essential oils and massage is its benefits to the muscles. It helps the body to keep it active and let it feel relaxed. Massage plays an important role on how essential oils can benefit your body. When it is massaged the right way, then there are endless benefits you can get from this.

These essential oils move through the body even by applying it. The oil penetrates to the body and travels to the body through the blood vessels. The best way to experience aromatherapy massage is inhaling the aroma into your body. It serves as a way of relaxing your body and making you feel good for yourself.

And since this is directly applied to the body, here are the benefits that you may get from aromatherapy for your muscles.

1. Aromatherapy helps improve the blood flow in your muscles by increasing the blood supply on your muscles which makes your muscles feel more nourished from the inside.
2. Massaging essential oils also relieves your muscles from painful and stiff feeling. A good massage and the use of essential oils can keep your muscles healthy and the circulation relieves of the pain and stiffness that you feel on your muscles.
3. Essential oils and massage also helps your connective tissue and muscles stretch well which improves your body's performance and allows you to do more activities that require stretching.
4. Essential oils make the body relaxed and same is true with your muscles. Applying essential oils helps relieve the sore feeling and prevents your muscles from feeling tight.

Benefits for your Skin and Hair

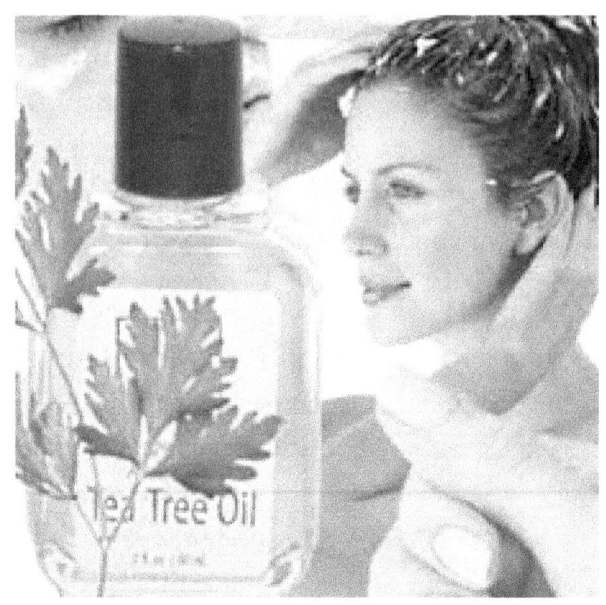

Essential oil applied directly on skin and hair gives a lot of benefits. This may include the following:

1. Get more moisturized skin. Essential oils helps lock in the moisture of your skin especially after bathing. This is the reason why applying this directly into skin can be very beneficial. Chamomile and lemon oil are noted for their properties of keeping your skin moisturized.

2. Essential oil applied on hair also helps keep it looking more alive. The reason for this is because it also locks in the moisture in your hair. This helps make your hair look more beautiful. Chamomile oil is known for making your hair moisturized.

3. Some essential oils prevent acne and pimple break outs and helps cure this skin conditions. The reason for this is because these oils contain antibacterial properties that help you get rid of these problems. Lavender oil is known to have these properties which helps fight these skin impurities. Also, tea

tree oil helps remove these skin conditions since they have antibacterial properties as well.

4. Some essential oils also helps promote skin regeneration and cell growth which improves the elasticity and flexibility of your skin. This helps avoid and reduce wrinkles and other skin impurities on your skin that is caused by aging. Noted oils that has this benefit is lavender oil and rose oil that keeps your skin firm. Sandalwood oil is also recognized as an effective oil for reducing wrinkles that most anti-aging products contain this oil.

5. Applying essential oils on your skin also helps you inhale the aroma which helps you to relax your mind and keeps you keep calm.

As you have read, essential oils can truly benefit your skin. Simply applying to your skin can already help treat a number of ailments and keep your skin moisturized. But there are other things that you should still know about aromatherapy and these health benefits will make you want to benefit from it.

THE HEART AND BLOOD CIRCULATION

Aside from its benefits to the skin and muscles, there are still several health benefits of essential oils to the body. The heart, in particular, benefits a lot in aromatherapy. This belief about the benefit of essential oils for the circulatory system has been there for quite a period of time and is one of the reasons why this alternative treatment has been used in Ayurvedic medicine.

1. The moment that you start aroma therapy, your heart starts to pump easier since this method releases stress and tension. Those who suffer from health problems like high blood pressure are advised to try this sine it helps blood to pump easily to the heart.

2. Since the heart gets energized with every sessions conducted, the heart becomes stronger. Lavender oils are noted for this ability.
3. There are essential oils that help unclog arteries whenever essential oils are applied to the location which makes widens it and makes it easier to open. If you want to benefit from this, then it is advisable for you to try applying juniper or rosemary oils to your skin.
4. If you are a person who has experienced heart failure in the past, then essential oil can help you prevent these episodes in the future. Camphor and peppermint oil are known to promote proper blood circulation to the heart without posing any risk to it. These oils actually help improve the function of your cardiac muscles if you have this problem in the past.

Aromatherapy and the Respiratory System

Just like the old saying goes "All Roads lead to Rome", same can be said about aroma therapy and the respiratory system. It is inevitable for you to inhale the aroma coming from this essential oil as you rub this or on your body or get a steam bath. Therefore, you benefit from aromatherapy with no extra effort.

You will be surprised about the number of benefits of aromatherapy to your respiratory that you'll really be amazed by this product.

1. Helps relieve Congestion- aromatherapy helps relieve congestion that is caused by blocked airways due to allergies. This can also be effective for those who are suffering from asthma. A mixture of rosemary, tea tree and hyssop can be used as an inhalant to relieve your nasal passages from congestion. It helps keep your airways open

and prevents congestion from occurring and becoming a burden to you.

The warm air that travels to your lungs during a steam bath or steam therapy can help you clear your airways which ease the clogged airways. The process triggers the bronchial passages to open which makes it easier for the air to get through the lungs and eventually makes breathing easier.

2. Coughing- when your throat feels itchy at times, this may cause you to cough due to the irritant that remains here. In order to stop the coughing, you may want to try anise and cypress oil in order to stop the inflammation in your throat and reduce the blockage in the area. Simply inhaling the vapors or steam from this oil is enough to keep you healthy which are the reason why it is no longer necessary for you to drink the solution.
3. Common Cold and Flu- since aromatherapy helps relax the respiratory system, it can also help reduce the duration of the symptoms of both common cold and flu. It can also reduce the inflammation caused by this illness by clearing out airways which makes those who suffer from these illnesses to feel eased.

There are thousands of essential oils if we are to consider the different sources their form. However, there are these noted oils that are renowned around the world for their overall benefits for the body. Here are the different oils that you should know and use in order for you to attain good health.

1. **Anise**- this is a very interesting plant since it is used in different industries. It is an herb that spoils quickly as soon as it is harvested so you should immediately extract the oil from the plant. Anise has a scent that is very similar like licorice. The scent is sweet and its oil is easy to use without any problems when it is inhaled. It can cure several problems that involve the respiratory system which may include bronchitis and asthma as well as relieve the common symptoms of cough and flu. It is important not to confuse this from star anise which is very similar to the regular anise when it comes to the scent and appearance but they both function differently.

2. **Basil**- according to researches, basil essential oils are good when it comes to dealing with feelings of fear, anxiety and even nervousness. It is even considered as the oil of "renewal" because of its properties. Basil has both strengthening and calming properties that is good to the heart and mind, which is good when you feel overwhelmed and stressed out. Some even claim that the oil from this plant helps overcome addiction. There are also bacteria that this oil inhibits which modern medicines find it hard to cure. Aside from these, it is said that basil is also good for rheumatism and other joint pains. Applying this on the swollen area can also relieve insect bites.

3. **Bergamot**- this fruit is found in many countries over the world and its oil is extracted for several medical purposes. It is also considered as one of the most favorite oil used in aromatherapy which is the reason why it is always on the list of essential oils that are purchased in the market. Here are the properties that makes bergamot one of the most sought essential oil:

- Antibacterial
- Anti-infectious
- Analgesic
- Anti-inflammatory
- Ant parasitic
- Antispasmodic
- Sedative
- Good for the digestive system.

Although this essential oil is often used to cure physical ailments, the digestive system and the skin in particular, it also promotes emotional wellness which is the greatest gift this citrus fruit has to offer.

4. The aroma of **birch oil** is very interesting since it doesn't contain the same "woody" scent like other tree oils. it smells more minty just like wintergreen. Also, it's properties and uses are the same with wintergreen. The way it helps cure the muscular and joint related problems is also similar to this plant. The reason for this is because both plants contain methyl salicylate, which may also act as an aspirin.

Other amazing properties of birch oil may include anti-inflammatory, antiseptic, antirheumatic, antispasmodic, analgesic, disinfectant, diuretic and stimulant. It also has warming properties that helps the skin adopt to the cold weather.

5. **Cedarwood**- the oil derived from this plant is frequently used for the nervous and respiratory system, although it also contains diuretic properties which benefits the urinary system as well. According to studies, the oil is high in sesquiterpenes, a plant compound to which researchers at the International Journal of Molecular Sciences believes to be effective in fighting human diseases.
Cedarwood essential oil benefits our mood and feelings as well. Cedarwood is said to have a calming effect on your nervous system and is even thought to have a special effect of uniting people together.

6. **Chamomile** most varieties of this plant have been used for centuries to calm your soul and assist you for a restful sleep, making it a popular oil to use before bed. Aside from that, there are other properties that are present in chamomile which benefits the body especualy when used in aromatherapy. This includes anti-parasitic, anti-infectious and anti-inflammatory properties that are good for the body.and as mentioned earlier, it has calming and relaxing effect which helps promote good sleep.

7. **Clove**- the oil derived from this plant can cure several diseases like cataract, hepatitis and herpes complex. It contains several properties like:
- Antibacterial
- Analgesic
- Antifungal
- Anti-inflammatory

- Anti-infectious
- Anti-tumor
- Anti-parasitic
- Anti-tumor
- Disinfectant

There are several researches that has proven that chamomile is proven to be effective in treating certain diseases like candida and cataracts. It can be applied directly on the skin or with a carrier oil like coconut oil. It is also very effective in treating toothache since the excruciating pain caused by this immediately vanishes as soon as this oil is applied on the affected area.

8. **Eucalyptus**- another oil that has a lot of benefits to the body is eucalyptus oil. The camp horous and slightly sweet aroma is known for its health benefit of the improving the condition of the respiratory system and other issues concerning it. It also helps solve skin and hair related concerns.

This oil can be applied topically but those with sensitive skin should first run a test since the oil may react to your skin. It can be diffused to the air through steam as well. Here are the following illnesses that eucalyptus oil treats.

- Asthma
- Bronchitis
- Diabetes
- Ear Inflammation
- Dysentery
- Emphysema
- Hypoglycemia

- Kidney Stones
- Measles

The oil is also known to be a good expectorant which drains the mucus from the lungs. It also cools the body when a person is having fever and helps regulate the body temperature.

9. **Frankincense**- the oil derived from this plant has been noted to be one of the most important essential oils there is. Who would forget that this is one of the gifts given to the Christ according to the gospel. If you'll read the benefits of this oil then you'll realize why this oil is precious during ancient times and even know.

According to studies, frankincense has been proven to help treat cancer through direct application on the reflex points of the body or of the feet or ingesting it by adding a drop of it on beverage. To prevent the muscles from atrophy, those who are on a state of coma are also massaged with this special oil on their hands and feet.

Other illnesses that this essential oil helps treat are the following:

- Coughs
- Depression
- Fibroids
- Genital Warts
- Hepatitis
- Infected Wounds
- Inflammation
- Liver Cirrhosis
- Lou Gehrig's Disease

10. **Ginger**- slightly sweet and slightly spicy oil is known to have an effect on the digestive system and the nervous system. As a matter of fact, other important health benefits of ginger oil is the effect it has on your mental, emotional, and spiritual health.

Here are the following diseases that ginger oil can help cure:

- Angina
- Club Foot
- Diarrhea
- Gas
- Indigestion
- Low Libido
- Pelvic Pain Syndrome
- Rheumatic Fever (Pain)
- Rheumatoid Arthritis
- Scurvy
- Vertigo

11. **Lavender**- this one of the most versatile oil since it helps treat a lot of diseases. It has a lot of beneficial properties like:

- Analgesic
- Anticonvulsant
- Antidepressant
- Anticoagulant
- Anti-infectious
- Antifungal
- Antihistamine
- Anti-inflammatory

- Antimicrobial
- Antimutagenic
- Antiseptic
- Antispasmodic
- Antitoxic

Although this essential oil may be very potent when it comes to combating diseases, it is actually one of the gentlest essential oil there is.

12. **Rosemary**- oil derived from this plant is also very beneficial and is proven to cure several diseases there is which includes the following:

- Adenitis
- Anxiety
- Arterial Vasodilator
- Arthritis
- Bell's Palsy
- Bronchitis
- Cancer
- Candida
- Cellulite
- Cholera
- Club Foot
- Colds
- Constipation
- Cough
- Dandruff
- Depression
- Diabetes
- Diuretic
- Fainting

- Fatigue
- Flu
- Hair Loss
- Headaches
- Inflammation
- Kidney Inflammation
- Low Blood Pressure
- Menstrual Irregularity
- Muscular Dystrophy
- Osteoarthritis
- Respiratory Infections
- Schmidt's Syndrome
- Sinusitis
- Staph Infections
- Strep Infections

Before applying this essential oil in your skin, it is important to check whether you are sensitive to the ingredients of this oil. Also, the use of this oil is prohibited for those who are pregnant or having epilepsy. it is also not advisable for the use of those who have high blood pressure.

13. **Tea tree**- the use of tea tree oil has been used in many cultures throughout history since and is commonly used to cure wounds. It is also believed that the oil has 12 times more antiseptic properties than phenol. This oil is both anti-fungal and antiviral which makes it good to treat those who are suffering from different infections. It's antiseptic properties helps clean and disinfect wounds effectively.

Here is a list of some of the diseases that tea tree oil helps cure

- Acne

- Aneurysm
- Athlete's Foot
- Boils
- Bacterial Infections
- Bronchitis
- Candida
- Chicken Pox
- Canker Sores
- Colds and Coughs
- Dermatitis
- Dry/Itchy Eyes
- Ear Infection/Ache
- Eczema
- Flu
- Fungal Infections
- Gum Disease
- Hepatitis
- Herpes Simplex
- Hives
- Infections (General)
- Inflammation
- Jock Itch
- Nail Infection
- Pink Eye
- Rashes
- Rubella
- Scabies
- Shingles
- Shock
- Sore Throat
- Staph Infection

- Sunburn
- Thrush
- Vaginal Infection
- Varicose Ulcer
- Viral Infections
- Warts

Carrier oils

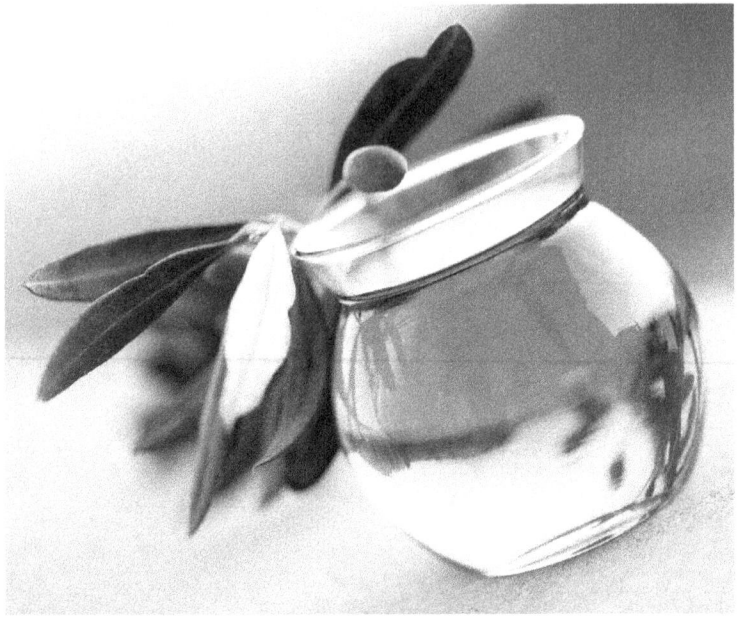

Most essential oils cannot stand alone and be applied directly into the skin. This is the reason why carrier oils are still necessary in order for you to use this kind of oil. These oils are commonly vegetable based oils taken from the fatty portion of plants, either from their seeds or kernel. These are oils to which essential oils are diluted before being applied on skin. Most of these oils already has their own health benefit but adding essential oils will make it more effective.

When considering on purchasing essential oils, it is important to consider the quality of the product that you want to purchase. Some essential oils get spoiled over time. Some last less than eight months depending on the ingredients they have.

There's quite a list for carrier oils and some of which are not really used frequently or are used only in specific situations this is the reason why we have included here the carrier oils that are commonly used along with essential oils.

Coconut oil

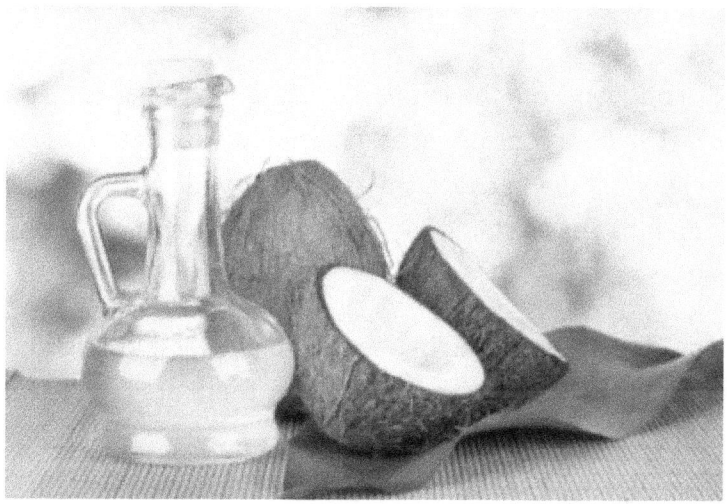

This oil alone is very effective in promoting good health. It is known to be an effective way of keeping your skin soft, silky and moisturized. It also promotes hair growth and keeps the hair manageable. This is the reason why most companies use this oil in their beauty products. It is no wonder then that coconut oil along with other essential oil is used to improve your skin's health.

In room temperature, coconut oil is solid. It is odorless and colorless which won't stain your clothes if you apply it on your skin. The main reason though why coconut oil is one of the most used carrier oil is its long shelf life. When added with other carrier oils, it also extends the shelf life of the product. Not to mention that the production of this oil has the lowest cost.

Almond oil

Oil that is used as carrier oil is almond oil which is derived from almond nuts. The oil comes out of the nut after being removed from its shell. The body easily absorbs it and leaves a sweet flavor in your skin.

Jojoba oil

This oil is derived from the jojoba plant and its oil makes up 50% of the seed. The oil is considered as a natural wax and is odorless. Its slight yellow tint won't cause any trouble to your clothes. This is another oil that has a stable shelf life and is liquid under room temperature.

Jojoba oil is easily absorbed by the skin and resembles the natural oil that occurs in it. This is the reason why there are people who prefer this over the other carrier oils there is.

Grapeseed oil

Another oil that is used as carrier oil is derived from grape seed. This is rich in antioxidants which is good not only for the skin but also for the body. Many considers it as an effective lubricant during massage and shaving.

The oil leaves a glossy film that protects the essential oils from evaporating. Saturation of this oil takes even longer than other carrier oils. There have been claims that this has astringent qualities that helps tone the skin and does not clog the pores.

Essential blends

In order for the skin and the body to benefit from the essential oils, it is important to dilute it on carrier oils. However, these essential oils can also be blended in order to come up with products that benefits the skin.

Here are a few samples of the essential blends that are frequently used in order to come up with products that benefit your health.

Anti-aging blend

Every one of us wants to achieve a youthful glow which is the reason why we seek ways on how to keep our skin younger looking. Essential oils promise you that achieving this kind of skin is possible. Here is a special blend for you to be able to attain younger looking skin.

Frankincense: helps cure age spots

Sandalwood: protects the skin from harmful UV Rays

Lavender: sooths irritated skin and burns.

Myrrh: great for chapped skin as well as skin infections.

Helichrysum: good for cell regeneration and protects the skin from the sun.

Rose: helps stop the breakdown of collagen that results to. It's considered as one of the best oils for the skin.

Bug Repellant

Another fascinating use of essential oil is its use as a bug repellant. We all know that there are illnesses that are caused by bugs which is the reason why it is wise to have a bug repellant handy. Essential oils are used to repel these blood sucking bugs and prevent you from getting sick. There are also properties that would even remove the itch caused by these bugs.

- Fractionated Coconut Oil

- Catnip Oil

- Amyris Oil

- African Sandalwood Oil

- Wild Orange Oil

- Fir Needle Oil

- Eucalyptus Oil

- Sandalwood Oil

- Rose Oil

- Citronella Oil

- Cedarwood Oil

All these oils help prevent bugs from coming near you since they are repelled by the scent coming from you. Of course, instead of repelling others, the scent of these oils would attract people instead with its very fragrant smell.

Detoxification blend

Detoxification is very important in order to get rid of the harmful substances that are in your body. This is the reason why detoxification is very important in order to cleanse your body from the toxins that are thriving inside it.

Essential oils can also help detoxify your body with its several herbs that are proven to get rid of these harmful chemicals and substances.

- Tangerine- the oil from this plant is known to benefit the digestive system

- Geranium- supports our hormonal system

- Juniper berry- helps the urinary system by flushing out the toxins in it.

- Rosemary oil- highly antioxidant and good for the digestive system

- Cilantro- known also to contain antioxidants and help flush heavy metals and lead from the body

Massage Blend

The blends mentioned earlier can be used as a massage. However, there is a specific blend that is best for massage.

Basil: relaxes the muscular system as well as the nervous system. Relieves with tension headaches as well

Grapefruit: helpful for stress and has a calming effect on the nervous system

Cypress: improves circulation and prevents cramps

Marjoram: Renowned for its support of muscle aches and pains, sprains, and joint concerns.

Lavender: Renowned for its impact on stress, pain, and its soothing properties to your muscles and joints. It also helps relieve your headache and tension.

Peppermint: Known to be helpful for cramps, muscle aches and pains. It has cooling effect in the body which makes it good for massage.

Skin Blend

For those who really want flawless skin free from acne and other impurities, here is a blend that is perfect for the skin.

Ho Wood: has an antiseptic property which is helpful in skin infections, and helps to revitalize the skin.

Tea Tree: renowned for its antibacterial, antifungal, and antiseptic. This also contains anti-inflammatory properties and speeds the healing process. This is a favorite among essential oils for eczema and other forms of dermatitis.

EucalytpusGlobulus: Anti-inflammatory, anti-infectious, anti-fungal and highly anti-bacterial.

Geranium: Sooths irritated skin

Litsea: the oil supports skin revitalization and contains antiseptic and antibacterial properties.

Black Cumin Seed Oil: contains high in levels of linoleic acid and speeds up wound healing while reduces pore blockage and impaction.

PRODUCTS IN THE MARKET

There are several blends that are already available in the market today which is the reason why you should not worry if you want to purchase a right blend for you. They are already made to apply and already contains the essential oils and carrier oils. All you need to do is massage or apply it to your skin.

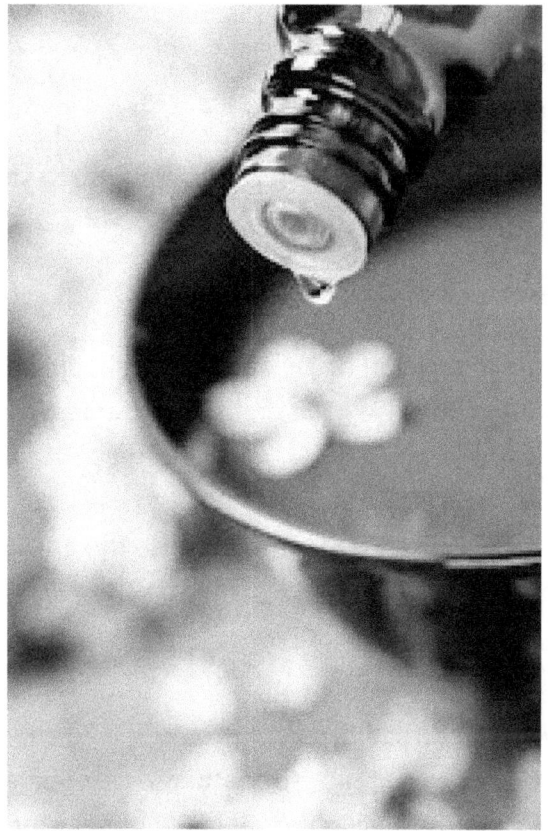

Those who want to practice aromatherapy should be aware that there are still several things to consider if you really want to practice this. There are several things to keep in mind from storing this special liquid on proper bottles to applying it to your skin. Here are some of the things that you still need to know about essential oils and aromatherapy.

Storage instructions:

It is highly advisable for you to use glass vials when it comes to storing your essential oils it is more effective in retaining the integrity of the liquid compared to plastic. It is also important to store this on blue or amber opaque vials to reduce the chances of sunlight from penetrating through the glass and affecting the quality of the product.

Store essential oils on cool place to keep its properties since warm temperatures decreases the quality. It is also wise to store it on a dark place to avoid exposure to sunlight.

Always dilute the oil

We keep on reminding you that essential oils should be diluted on carrier oils like the ones we have mentioned earlier. There are instances that your skin may be sensitive to these oils when it is applied as it is. The truth is that it is better to use just a little amount of this oil and it doesn't compromise the quality of the product you have.

Do A check up

Before applying this directly on your skin, it will be good if you try a patch test in order to see if the aromatherapy products you'll use will be safe for you. This will help you know if the oil poses any risk to your skin that may damage it.

Do not ingest the product

It's not because we have discussed that this product is all natural that you should swallow these oils or take it orally. It is very important to seek advice from your doctor first before taking in anything.

Use for Children

It is alright to use a little of these essential oils to children but it is important to remember to use only very little amount of this oil on the affected area. This is to avoid some serious problems that may be caused by using these oils.

Ask Your Doctor

Talk to your doctor about using these essential oils and going through aroma therapy. The doctor knows your medical history and could say whether this procedure or alternative medicine will be good for your body or not considering your overall health.

Conclusion

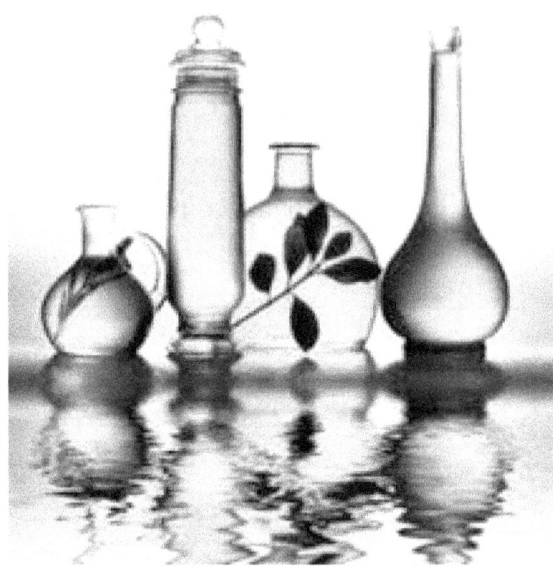

As you will notice, there are several advantages of aromatherapy to the body. It is truly an effective way of promoting good health and helps treat some of the illnesses and diseases we have in the body.

It is one of the most interesting form of treatment there is for several diseases that are prevalent today. We also have understood why aromatherapy can benefit your overall health.

You should take a look at aromatherapy when you are finding ways to make it easier for your body to feel its best. Aromatherapy can be used with all sorts of essential oils that have their own natural properties and many other features. These include carrier oils that will help you out with giving your body a better sense of control.

The world of essential oils is very interesting and amusing. They are made from different ingredients that can be beneficial for whatever result you want to achieve. Aromatherapy is made to improve your health.

The methods used in aromatherapy also vary and you may choose among the choices what to employ and this depends upon the need and the capacity of your body. You may even try all methods at home every once in a while.

Aromatherapy is believed to be one of the most effective treatments there is for several diseases and ailments. This is the reason why it is still popular to this day. There are several oils that you can choose from if you truly are interested in trying this to assist in curing whatever ailment you have or just to keep yourself calm.

What really matters is to follow closely what is rewritten on this guide in order to get the full benefits of aromatherapy. This way, you'll feel a lot healthier while in the comfort of your very home.

www.ingramcontent.com/pod-product-compliance
Lightning Source LLC
Chambersburg PA
CBHW071140280526
45787CB00003B/1357